DR. PRADNYA SRIRAM

the STETHOSCOPE AROUND MY NECK

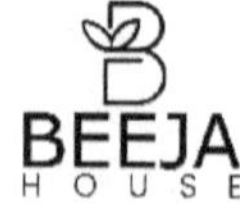

Copyright © 2023 **Dr. Pradnya Sriram**

ISBN: 978-93-95266-72-7

Published by: Beeja House

Printed By: Repro India Ltd.

First Printing Edition 2023

Author Email: pradnyasriram13@gmail.com

Dedicated to my teacher, the Late Dr. Shirolkar

To my parents, Arvind and Chitra Vaidya

To my beautiful daughters, Divya and Shreeya

*To my husband, Dr. Sriram Ramalingam, who has been
a constant support*

Prologue

This book is about Dr. Padma and the challenges she faces in her career as an anaesthesiologist

An anaesthesiologist has been denied due recognition in India. The career of an anaesthesiologist is very challenging as they thread the fragile line between life and death. There is no room for error as it could cost the life of the patient.

I am sure you will enjoy the book as you embark on the Anaesthesia journey along with Dr. Padma.

The case scenarios are real as they are the author's personal experiences. The names of the characters have been changed but the hospital names have been retained

Contents

Chapter One

When The Patient Almost Died

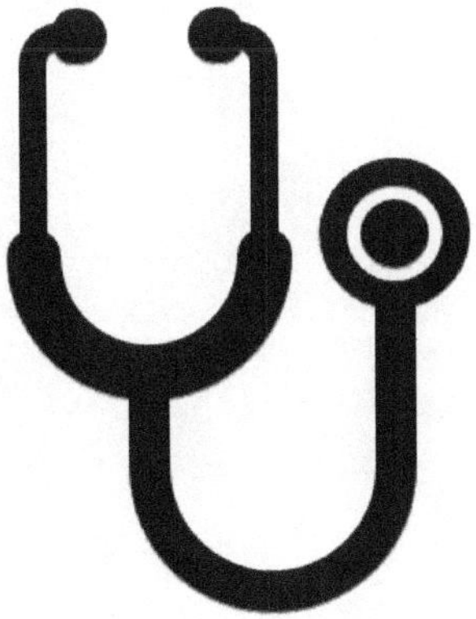

The trainee nurse came running towards operation theatre number two and called out frantically, "The caesarean patient had a cardiac arrest in operation theatre number one."

The trainee nurse trembled. She had never experienced a situation like this. Her petite body was drenched in sweat. The situation was serious and needed Dr. Padma's attention immediately. Dr. Padma was the anaesthesiologist on-call that day and she was responsible for all the emergency cases on her on-call day.

It was a routine emergency day. The emergency was as heavy as any other day with patients piling up as usual. The hospital was a government hospital and this was expected. The corridors of the Emergency OPD wing were hustling with all kinds of people from injuries to pain to fever. The staff was doing their best to manage the crowd. Some of the doctors were working beyond their duty hours.

Padma had not changed out of her OT Attire that she had adorned in the morning for her routine day at the operation theatre as she had to continue from her routine cases to the emergency cases. The last case on the list was supposed to be over in some time. The sister in-charge, Sister Heilda, came in and handed over the emergency register to Padma. Sister Heilda smiled and said to Dr. Padma, "Long list already. Don't know how the on-call will unfold? You better go girl and grab something to eat. You don't know when you will find time later."

Sister Heilda was an Anglo-Indian lady in her fifties. She was a tall person, heavily built. She was beautiful, well-dressed in her gown and commanded respect. Sister Heilda was very good at her work and was overall in charge of the operation theatres. All doctors respected her. She was a motherly figure who was always ready to help but was very strict when it came to duty. The senior most doctors, too, had no say when it came to her rules.

Padma was already visualising her day. She had to prioritise all the cases for emergency surgeries according to their urgency. She knew it was to be a heavy emergency night. There was an emergency caesarean case that would always be on the top of the priority list. She also had a 1-year-old child's case, who needed immediate attention. Padma had already informed the emergency OT staff of these two cases and asked them to get the theatres ready. She had decided that her junior Dr. Shama would attend to the caesarean case. Dr. Shama was good and handled caesarean cases well. On the insistence of Sister Heilda, she did manage to eat something on the go. Padma looked smart in the green trousers and shirt and with a stethoscope around her neck. Of course, she managed all her cases with confidence.

Two operation theatres were running simultaneously. Padma's emergency days were always busy. Her juniors who were posted under her considered her jinxed. That meant the days they were on call with Padma they too would have a busy emergency night. But Padma thought it was a great opportunity to learn and was happy to soak up the knowledge and experience she got when she was on call and so did she tell her juniors.

Padma was busy with a paediatric case of a 1-year-old child with severe stomach pain. The child was a slum dweller's son. He was malnourished and writhing in pain. She felt sorry for the child and quickly put him to sleep by inducing anaesthesia. It was a difficult case. The child was vomiting frequently and there was a danger that some of the fluid could enter his lungs which would then make the situation critical. Padma looked at the child. A tiny little boy was lying listlessly on the operation table. The surgeon and his assistant had already started the surgery. The bright light was focused on the patient's abdomen. They were trying to find the cause of the obstruction. The only sounds heard in the theatre were of the pulse beats on the ECG monitor and the sound of the gases coming out of the anaesthesia bag.

The surgeon was suspecting a blockage in the intestine due to worms and his clinical judgement was accurate. Padma thought, "How could this little frame of the body have so many worms in it? What is life for these people who live on the streets? What could be the child's future?"

The surgery had just started and all seemed fine till the frantic call by the trainee nurse from the other operation theatre broke the calm.

Dr. Padma looked at sister Janaki, summoned her in, and said, "Take the bag and keep pressing." She knew sister Janaki was a senior experienced nurse with over 10 years of experience. It was her day off. She was packing up after her day assisting with the routine cases and was about to leave. But assessing the situation Sister Janaki immediately volunteered to help.

Padma was handing over the anaesthesia bag that is practically the child's life to her, but she had no choice. The Surgeon and Dr. Padma exchanged glances. He said, "You go and I will take care of the child." Padma then hurried to Operation theatre 2.

"What happened?" she asked. The ECG monitor showed a flat line. Her junior was already doing chest compressions. Everyone was in a state of panic mode. There was a bemused expression on everyone's face. Emergency drugs were being loaded. Padma took control of the situation. There the mother lay on the operation table listless and the baby had not been delivered. "Deliver the baby quickly!" Padma called out to the Obstetrician. Although Padma was a well-experienced anesthesiologist, each case was different. Her heart was pumping so fast that she could actually hear it. But at that very moment, all she wanted to hear was the patient's heart beats. Prayer on her lips she was doing everything possible to save the patient. The Obstetrician was already at his job. Suddenly everyone heard the cry of the baby and it was music to their ears. "Is the baby OK," Padma asked and in the same breath shouted out to the mother, "You better come back to hold your baby girl."

It was a shout of desperation. The ECG monitor beeped and beeped again. Was it God's grace or Dr. Padma's commitment that saved the mother, no one knows? One thing Padma learned through her experience is never to give up.

Have you ever thought about this? Why does this happen that in a state of desperation, everything begins to take a U-turn to happen the right way? Have you experienced this? There is a saying that failure is a stepping stone to success. Is it? Give it a thought. You must have read that most of the successful people had a desperate movement before they picked up their reins and stormed the world with their success stories. What did they do differently that the others didn't? Why don't all the people out there who have been desperate see a miracle if you want to call it so? Were the successful just lucky?

It's just that they called to God or the universe whatever you may call it from the bottom of their heart and asked for help. It's when the frequency of their calling matched God's frequency so that God could hear them. It's just like tuning into the right radio station to hear your favourite song. The frequencies have to match correctly or there will be a disturbance. These miracles do happen in a doctor's life and the doctors actually have a term for it "GOD ONLY KNOWS"

Three minutes had passed by. There was silence followed by claps and rejoicing. Dr. Padma had saved the mother. Padma monitored the patient for some time, ensured that she had recovered well, and then gave instructions to shift the patient to the ICU and rushed back to the operation theatre number two where she sent her junior Dr. Shama to manage the case. As she entered everyone looked up. Padma gestured a thumbs up. The surgery of the child was going on well. Dr. Shama was in tears when she saw Dr. Padma. Padma first thanked Nurse Janaki for her support and gestured a thank you to the surgeon too. Dr. Padma looked at Shama, "Don't worry we will discuss the case later. I will have to report to our HOD tomorrow but don't be scared, I will stand by you. This is a part of your learning process and you now know how to manage a situation like this. "The words she had just said resonated in her mind. All this brought back memories of the past when she had almost decided to quit the department two years back...

Department Of Anaesthesia

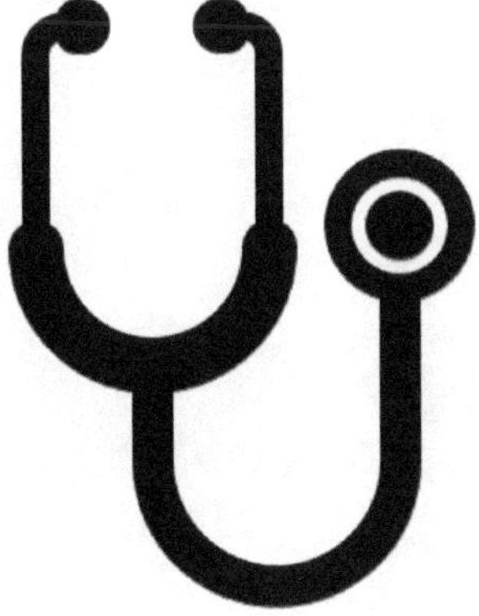

Dr. Padma was 15 days old in the department of anaesthesia. She was happy that she had chosen anaesthesia and was looking forward to the 3 years of residency. The department of anaesthesia was on the 6th floor of the JJ Hospital. This magnificent hospital has stood the test of time. Its history goes way back to 1845 when Sir Jamshedji Jeejeebhoy came forward with a donation of rupees one lakh for the establishment of a hospital. The inauguration took place on May 15, 1845. The foundation stone of Grant Medical College was laid on March 30, 1843, by Sir Robert Grant and it was opened on November 1, 1845, admitting the first batch of eight students. JJ Hospital has three peripheral hospitals, the St George's Hospital, the Cama and Albless Hospital, and the G.T Hospital, all located near the then V.T. station now the Sri Chhatrapati Shivaji station. Grant Medical College has produced a galaxy of eminent doctors and medical teachers and made its place on the world map. Reita Faria, Miss World 1966 and Aditi Govitrikar, Mrs. World 2001 are GMC Alumni.

But something was to change today. Padma was posted in the Cama and Albless Hospital, the famous government hospital in Bombay (now Mumbai) for mother and child care. It was her first posting. Her senior was Dr. Sheeba, a strict anaesthesiologist who could be very mean to her juniors. She was short and dark, and always had a frown on her face. She was good at her work and loved to throw her weight around. One could be either in her good books or very bad books.

That day Dr. Padma was all excited to see her first epidural anaesthesia. She had done her homework and read up all about it. It is a type of anaesthesia like spinal anaesthesia which is given in the spine and requires expertise. Since it's a blind procedure one needs to have a good experience. The patient was a tall, heavily built lady. She was posted for medical termination of pregnancy followed by tubal ligation as she didn't want any more children. She already had two daughters and one son.

Padma was surprised when Dr. Sheeba, after injecting 10 ml of the drug, summoned her to inject the remaining 10 ml of the drug. Padma was nervous and thought it was not right to do it as she had no experience but she couldn't voice her thoughts. Dr. Padma had hardly injected 2 ml of the drug when the patient collapsed. Dr. Sheeba took over immediately shouting instructions to Padma to load the syringes for the emergency drugs. Dr. Sheeba saved the patient but Padma was in tears. She got a sound hearing from her senior and was accused of the mishap. Padma had been instructed to monitor the patient all night. "We have to meet our HOD first thing in the morning, "Dr. Sheeba shouted as she left the ward. Dr. Padma had overheard her senior complaining to the ward nurse in charge, "We would have lost the patient today. I don't trust her, keep an eye on the patient. Being an anaesthetist is not a joke. It is one of the toughest branches for specialisation. I don't know why such people should take up this speciality." Dr. Sheeba's words exploded with eccentric nastiness. Padma had felt miserable and had made up her mind to quit the department. Padma diligently monitored the patient the whole night. The patient had a severe headache and was shouting and writhing in pain. The patient was given a head-low position to prevent excessive leakage of the spinal fluid. Dr. Padma felt miserable and blamed herself for the patient's sorry state.

Dr. Shirolkar the head of the department of anaesthesia was not only a great teacher but also a gentleman. The budding anaesthesiologist who trained under his tutelage received a clear knowledge of the subject. He was short with a receding hairline and was an authority in his subject who would always encourage his students. Some things which he taught left a permanent imprint in Padma's mind. He always told his students, "Anaesthesia is one field where the line between life and death is very fine. Please take a few seconds to confirm the drug before you inject it because once you inject a drug you cannot retrieve it if you have made an error. The surgeon can always redo the surgery if he makes a mistake but you cannot. There is no scope of if and but in our speciality."

He asked Dr. Sheeba and Dr. Padma to be seated. Padma was very nervous. She was sitting at the edge of the chair. Her heart was beating fast and her palms were cold and clammy. She wanted to rehearse the answers to the probable questions but her mind had gone blank. Just then she heard Dr. Shirolkar's voice. "Yes, tell me what happened," he asked Dr. Sheeba. Dr. Sheeba narrated the events of the previous day and blamed Dr. Padma for the total spinal. It's so called as the brain also gets anaesthetised in this complication which may cause the heart and lungs to stop working. Sheeba then added, "Sir, because of my expertise and God's grace I have saved the patient. It would have become a big issue as she was a patient for a family planning procedure." Padma was chagrined and in tears. She felt that Dr. Sheeba seemed to derive some kind of sadistic pleasure while blaming her for the incident. Dr. Shirolkar looked at Dr. Padma and consoled her. "Drink some water," he said. Dr. Shirolkar continued, "Why are you crying? You should consider yourself lucky to have managed a total spinal. Many of my resident doctors will not see or manage this complication in their three years of residency. More the complications you see in your residency days, the better and more confident anaesthesiologist you will be." Something in his words struck a chord. Padma soon felt at ease. He then looked at Dr. Sheeba and said, "Don't you think it's too early to allow a 15-day-old resident to give epidural anaesthesia. It's your mistake. We will discuss this case in the morbidity mortality meeting. You both may leave now." This was a total turn of events. Padma was not expecting this. She knew now that she was in a good department headed by an excellent head of department. She didn't want to quit but she also knew she would have to cross roads with Dr. Sheeba during her residency period and now she was in her very bad books.

Cama Hospital's posting was to be a very memorable posting for Dr. Padma as it was also the place where she was reborn.

Chapter Three

Rebirth

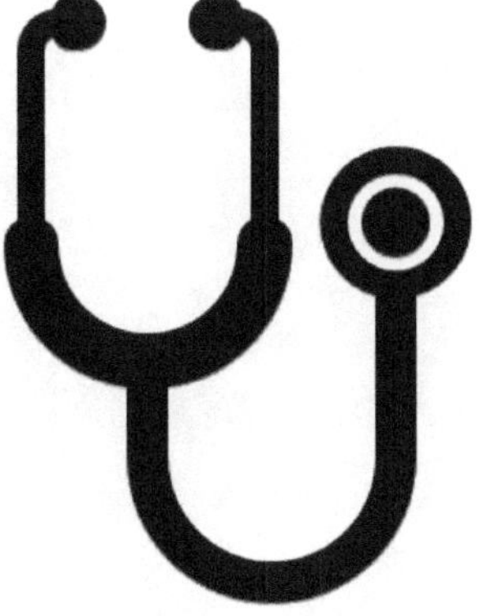

It was June 6, 1991. The Bombay rains had as in all years unleashed their fury. The monsoon in Bombay is well-known for its torrential rains and could cause water logging everywhere. Every year at least it would be 2 days when a city like Bombay that never sleeps would come to almost a standstill.

Mumbai is made of seven islands and has a long history behind it. It is not only the financial capital of India but also has the eighth-highest number of billionaires. It is not only known for Bollywood but also has Asia's largest slum called Dharavi. Mumbai is popularly seen to be a city that shelters and feeds all. Mumbai's social fabric is there to see. There is a wide gap between the rich and the poor. It's like two distinct cities exist within one. There are the houses of the famous Bollywood actors facing the Sea and then your gaze couldn't miss the slums by the same sea shore. All things apart Mumbai does have a charisma of its own. The energy is palpable.

Bombay has a special place in Padma's heart. It was the city where Padma was born and today, she will be born again.

Padma had been on her emergency call the previous night. She was asked to continue the next day too as it was near to impossible for anyone to travel in these torrential rains. Dr. Jitu was her senior that day. He was not only an excellent anaesthesiologist but also a considerate and honest person. He was a great teacher and would always encourage his juniors with positive words. "Padma, you will manage the case today, "he said. "You shall tell me your anaesthesia plan. See to it that all the syringes including the emergency drugs are loaded and labelled." Dr. Padma managed the general anaesthesia case well under Dr. Jitu's supervision. It was time to get the patient out of anaesthesia. Dr. Jitu asked Padma to get the suction machine to the head end of the patient. It was needed to suck the secretions in the patient's throat when the patient would be coming out of anaesthesia.

Padma switched on the machine and pulled the machine with her right hand and she collapsed. When she became aware of her surroundings, she could hear her name being called out and was being asked about her well-being. Padma tried to get up but felt weak in her right leg. Dr. Jitu asked her to lie down. She could feel that an IV line was put in her left hand. She was confused and asked, "What happened?" Dr. Jitu reassured her and said, "You were almost electrocuted when you pulled the suction machine. Looks like a short circuit because of the rain."

What a change of fate, a moment of sheer serendipity, the emergency injections which she had loaded for the patient were being used for her. It was a routine practice for an Anesthetist to keep some basic emergency drugs loaded and labelled on their anaesthesia machine in case the need arises. And today it saved Padma's life.

She was still trying to get hold of the situation when the ward boys came with the stretcher to shift her to the ICU in the main JJ Hospital. It took some time to reach the hospital. Although there was no traffic, the roads were completely flooded. The rains had not taken a breather. Dr. Padma was shifted onto the stretcher and was hand-lifted down the stairs. The ambulance was already waiting at the hospital entrance. They then shifted Padma to the ambulance. She felt miserable and just wanted to run away. Could she at least sit up but she was strictly instructed to lie down? Doctors indeed make the worst patients. The ambulance moved at a very slow pace. There was water logging everywhere. Dr. Padma's classmate Dr. Sirisha. a gynaecology resident was accompanying her. As they entered gate 5 of J.J hospital, Dr. Sirisha called out to Dr. Ram who was waiting at the gate. Ram and Padma had been together for the last 3 years. Marriage was on the cards for the next year. Ram had to wade through the knee-deep water to reach the ambulance. He saw the bewildered look on Padma's face and the tears in her eyes. He held her hand and said, "Don't worry. You will be fine. "At the main building, the elevator was shut off. Water had entered the ground floor of JJ hospital. The usually crowded OPD looked a bit deserted. But the doctors were still busy attending to emergencies wading through the water-logged floor.

The stretcher had to be again lifted to the ICU which was on the 5th floor. Padma felt sorry for the ward boys and kept insisting that she could walk up but her words fell on deaf ears. Physically also she wouldn't have been able to as her right leg felt weak.

Padma was wheeled into the ICU. At the ICU she was connected to the ECG monitor. There is a possibility of arrythmias which is an erratic rhythm of the heart to occur after electrocution. The cardiologist examined her and said, "You are fine Dr. Padma but we will have to keep you for observation for 48 hours. "Looking at the bewildered look on Padma's face he smiled, "You are fine now but we cannot take chances. Arrythmias are known to occur after electrocution. Do you know that your heart had almost stopped to a heart rate of 20? Thanks to Dr. Jitu, you are alive today," the cardiologist said. Padma thought, "Really, was it so bad? Looks like it's my rebirth and Dr. Jitu my God father." Padma thanked God for everything. But she was upset about her predicament to stay in the ICU for 48 hours. Did she have a choice? 24 hours had passed uneventfully. Padma had managed her night in the ICU but with little sleep. She felt bad that she was occupying a precious bed in the ICU. JJ Hospital was a government hospital and so was free of charge. There was always an overload of patients and which meant there must be a waiting list to avail of the ICU facilities. So, she decided to convince the cardiologist to discharge her and she would stay for the next 24 hours in her friend's room, a radiology resident who was on the same floor. She was successful.

Padma had insisted that her family should not be informed but the damage had already been done. As a protocol, her aunt who was her local guardian had been informed. That meant her parents were informed and her father would be already on the way to Bombay from Pune. Padma knew her father would be very apprehensive and would be eager to meet her. She could reminisce about the day when she got her admission to the medical college and the joy on her dad's face. Her maternal grandfather was so proud of her. He always wanted his first-born grandchild to be a doctor and study in the same college, the Grant Medical College where he also had studied and so had her uncle and aunts. They were all GMCites as anyone from Grant Medical College is called.

Chapter Four

Childhood Days

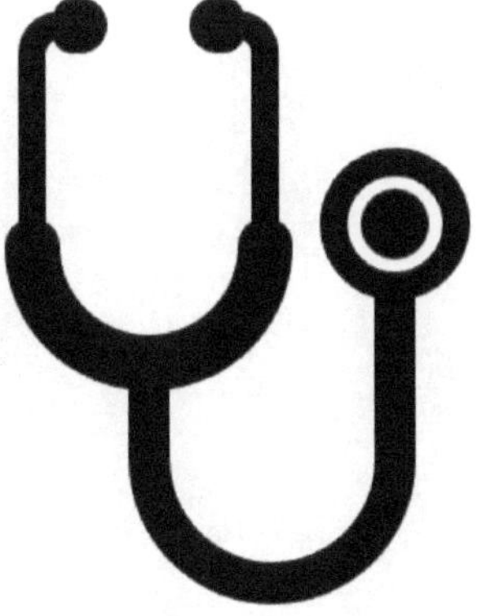

Padma's thoughts drifted to the early days and her journey of becoming a doctor. The seed of her passion to become a doctor was sowed very early in her childhood. She came from a family of doctors. Her grandfather and her aunts and uncles all were doctors. As a child, she had already made up her mind. Padma had stayed with her maternal grandparents during her early school days. She remembered the day when her grandfather had decided to take her along with him to Bombay and get her admitted to a new school. This situation had arisen because of certain circumstances. Dr. Padma's father, an Airforce officer was posted at Hyderabad. Padma was admitted to the first standard in a school that was close to their house. It was the month of December when her grandfather had come to Hyderabad for a medical conference. He happened to go to the school to pick up his granddaughter and was surprised to see little Padma sitting in a large room with other kids who seemed to be of all age groups. He later learned that all primary classes were combined in one room for want of classrooms in a government school. He was upset and that's when he decided to take Padma to Bombay. Padma stayed in Bombay at her grandfather's house till she completed her second grade. She was pampered by all. Her aunts and uncles made sure that Padma would not miss her parents. After all, she was just a child.

Time flew by and it was time to be back in Hyderabad with her parents and sisters and in a new school. She was flying alone from Bombay to Hyderabad on Indian Airlines. Padma was only 5 years old and as a protocol, she was to be in the care of an Air Hostess and her father would come to receive her from the aircraft at Hyderabad. She was bold and actually enjoyed her flight. By the time she landed in Hyderabad her little purse was full of chocolates that were given to her on the flight.

Padma was excited about being back home with her sisters and parents. She was also looking forward to joining the new school. It was a newly commissioned Kendriya Vidyalaya. Padma remembered the day she went for the school interview. She was seeking admission to the third grade. Her father, who was a very disciplined and meticulous person, had made sure that his daughter was dressed in a pretty frock and had polished black shoes on with matching socks to go. Padma looked smart. Padma's father had also made sure that all the required documents were neatly placed in a folder and labelled. These meticulously organised documents helped Padma not only get admission but also she became the first student of the school. Her admission number was one. Actually, Padma was second in line for the admission process. The child who first went into the principal's office didn't have her papers right and so Padma was called in for admission. Padma loved to go to school. She was made the class leader for 4 consecutive years. She always dressed well and was well-mannered. Mannerism and discipline were inculcated naturally into her and her sisters. After all, she was a defence personnel's daughter. The etiquettes, table manners, and discipline were all taught to them since their early childhood.

Padma was immersed in her thoughts of her childhood days. Padma had just then come back from school. She was let in by the housemaid Fatima. Fatima took the school bag from Padma and went in. Padma heard her mother call out from the kitchen, "Today I have made some chat items. Go quickly, have a wash, change your clothes and come." Padma knew the routine. She had to first take off her shoes and socks and place them on the shoe rack. Then after a hand and face wash, she had to change into a fresh set of home clothes. She had to make sure she had hung her uniform on the hanger and place it in its designated place. Although Padma's household had servants to take care of all their needs, all three sisters were taught not to totally depend on the servants. It was something that helped Padma in the long run.

Fatima and her family worked in Padma's house. They lived in the servant quarters. Fatima was one of three siblings. She had an elder brother and an elder sister. They lived with their parents. Her brother had a job as a mechanic and their father had no job. The women worked in Padma's house. Fatima was 18 years old. But she was still like a child and loved to play with Padma and her sisters. She looked after them and gave them company when Padma's parents would have to attend parties. She was average-built and always had a smile on her face. Then one evening Fatima's mother along with her two daughters came with a box of sweets and proudly announced that she had found grooms for her daughters. Fatima's sister Zareen was just a year and a half older than Fatima. Padma's mother asked about the alliance and was aghast to know they were being married off to some Sheikhs in Saudi who were forty years old. Padma's mother tried to dissuade the girls' mother and told her not to get them married so soon. She tried to convince her to get them married to someone younger and from India. But it was in vain as the parents had been offered money and gifts by the Sheikhs. Everything was arranged and the girls had to fly the next month. Padma was in the eighth grade then. She felt bad for Fatima who was still naïve and childish. After all, money could buy anything and another reason that Fatima's mother gave was that the girls would be safe once they were married. Was Fatima's mother being delusional? The sad truth was Fatima was just going to be another addition to the Sheikh's harem. She bore a child for him every year. The last Padma heard about Fatima was when she was already a mother of 5 children in 6 years.

Padma's school days were joyful and her childhood was carefree and protected. She continued her education in Hyderabad till the 10th standard and again went back to Bombay to realise her dream.

Becoming A Bombayit

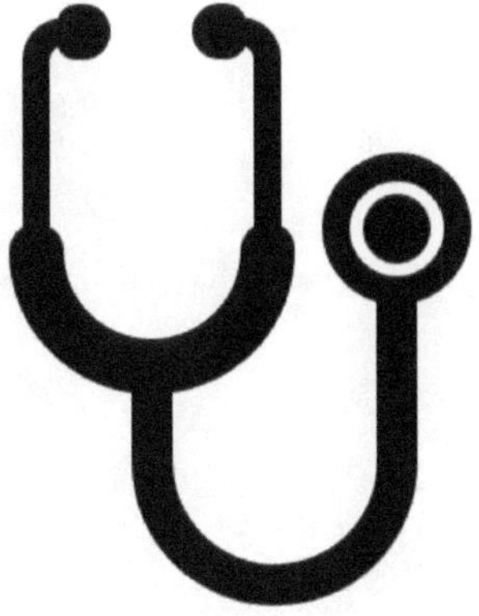

Padma's journey to becoming a doctor had already started at her grandparents' house and as days went by her determination grew even stronger. She was back in Bombay after her 10th grade to seek admission to a Bombay college. It was a prerequisite that she had to pass her 12th board exams from Bombay to get admission to a medical college there. Her father came to leave Padma at her grandfather's house. This was the beginning of the second phase of her journey to becoming a doctor and to an adventurous life in the city called Bombay, now Mumbai. It was a stark difference to live a life in a city like Bombay from the protected life she had lived with her parents. When she first came to Bombay for education, she was a child and everything was taken care of but now the situation was different. Padma realised that there would be no one to hand hold now and she would have to learn to live the Bombay way on her own. It was especially difficult for her because she came from a very protected environment. Padma had never travelled by public transport. It was a big learning curve to travel by bus and most importantly by the local trains, the life lines of Bombay. Luckily, she was a Maharashtrian and knew the local language. Not that one has to learn Marathi to survive in Mumbai. It's a cosmopolitan city where people from all over India come to live their dreams. It's a city of opportunities.

Padma had secured admission in Mithibai College at Vile Parle. Vile Parle, famous for its Parle biscuits, was the next station stop after Andheri. Andheri was the suburb where Padma's grandparents lived. The concept of local trains was completely new to her. This ignorance got her into trouble on the very first day of her journey back from college. No one had told her that there were trains that would have their last destination as Andheri and some trains, although stopping at Andheri would continue their onward journey. Why was this so important, especially for a newcomer? The veterans, the so-called Bombayits, now Mumbaikars would appreciate it. Travelling by local trains is an art by itself which every Mumbaikar knows and the newcomers eventually learn it. Two things Padma learned that day were that one has to be very quick and smart to travel by the locals and that timing is all that counts.

Padma that day had her worst experience. She climbed into, or it would be appropriate to say, she was pushed in at the Parle station along with the other ladies. Even before she could settle down, her destination had arrived in a few minutes. Padma was unaware that she should have moved to the entrance of the compartment to get down at the next station. Padma tried to get out at the Andheri station but before she could climb down, she was pushed back in again by the incoming crowd. She tried to wriggle out shouting that she wanted to get out. Suddenly she was pushed by someone onto the platform. Before she could realise what had happened the train had already left the station. There was soon a crowd of new faces awaiting the next train oblivious of her plight. A good

Samaritan helped her to stand up and collect her belongings. She smiled at Padma and said, "Looks like you are new to Bombay. Don't worry, you will soon learn." Padma at the end of this horrifying ordeal had a torn dress and a shattered mind. But soon she overcame her fears and became a veteran.

Bombay locals are unique. They are always on time and most of the time overcrowded especially during the peak hours. They engulf a world of their own. The ladies' compartment revealed some interesting anecdotes every time she travelled in it. There were women of all ages and attitudes. There were children going to or coming back from school chatting, eating, or playing some games oblivious of their surroundings. You might also see a helpful lady offering her seat to an elderly woman. You might also see women rushing in jostling their way to catch a seat, not ashamed to push a mother with a child who would have to stand throughout the journey. Maybe another woman would offer to take the child from the standing mother for some time and make the baby sit on her lap. Then there would be women and children selling bangles, hair clips, bindis, and other things. One could see vendors selling vegetables. Some passengers would buy from them and also in fact cut them and put them in small boxes or covers. These ladies would come prepared with the things needed to prep the veggies for their dinner or the next day's lunch. Life in Bombay ran by the clock and time management was so crucial. All Bombayits take life with a stride and Padma had to do the same.

 Padma had decided to face all challenges with grit for her only aim was to become a doctor. Life in Bombay was to teach her many things. She could no longer be naïve. She had to become street-smart and she did.

Padma's pre-med days were interlaced with interesting situations, be it having to learn to travel in Bombay or deal with eve teasing. Also, she learned the art of studying in a chaotic environment of small spaces combined with noise pollution from the blaring sounds of loud speakers playing some Bollywood numbers. She was literally living out of bags. Padma had to shift residence to her aunt's place for four months when her grandparents had to visit her uncle in the US. She was a very accommodating person and managed well in any place or circumstance. By now she had become a Bombay girl. Padma continued to focus on her studies. Time flew by so fast that it was already time for the 12th board exams. She was burning the midnight oil and she had to again make peace with the new situation that had arisen just a few months before her finals. It was her uncle's wedding and she somehow sailed through the chaotic days of a wedding house.

At last, the day Padma was waiting for dawned was full of hope. It was the day she would get admission to the famous Grant Medical College. Her father was with her during the admission and he felt so proud of her.

It was a joyous moment that she shared with her grandparents and her family. It would be the beginning of a new inning in her life. The journey had just begun.

MBBS Days

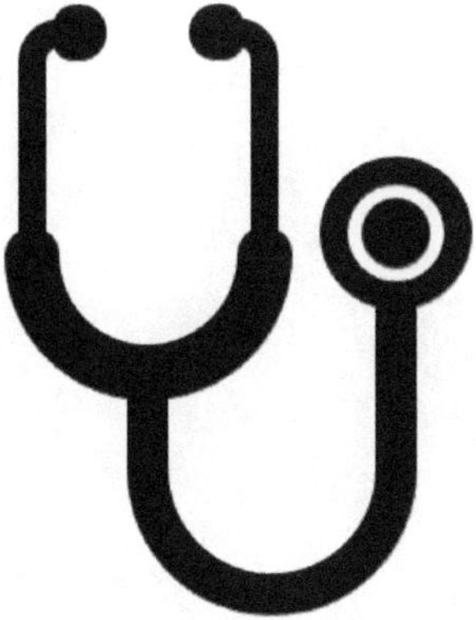

The new batch of 1984 had assembled in the famous Anatomy Hall of the Grant Medical College. This was the same hall that was featured in the movie *Munna Bhai MBBS*. It was a huge hall with a semi-circular wooden table in the front. All were happy but also anxious about the ragging that would soon follow in the coming weeks. It was a part and parcel of the MBBS days. Padma's batch had managed to escape the first ragging and so the whole batch was subjected to a mass ragging by the seniors at the same Anatomy Hall full of vengeance. They all were made to dance on the table of the Anatomy Hall and take an oath with all the medical jargon which they hardly understood then. Actually, if one could translate the oath into spoken English, it would be censored. The ragging didn't end there but continued for some more days in both hostels: ladies and men.

Padma, being an out-stationed candidate, eventually stayed in the Ladies' Hostel throughout her MBBS years. The freshers for the first 6 months had to stay in the terrace room which was also nicknamed the 'Hawa Mahal'. It was a huge room that could accommodate at least 12 girls. It opened to the terrace which was a meeting place for the girls. One could see the other buildings on the campus. The terrace was also big enough to accommodate a lot of pigeons that would go about with their own activities oblivious of girls who were standing in groups chatting and gossiping. They shared the space rather amicably.

Then suddenly one could hear the voice of the watchman shouting out the name of one of the hostel girls three times to notify her that she had a visitor. It would be an utter embarrassment for the poor girl especially when she didn't want the other girls to know about her boyfriend. Alas, she couldn't escape the inquisitive and peering eyes of the girls looking down from the terrace or from the windows of their rooms to know who this visitor was.

The terrace room had no furniture. They had to get their bedding which was put on the floor and all their belongings were stacked up in their suitcases. It was the time all the hostilities from the new batch would get ragged but eventually, these very seniors became their good friends who guided and helped them. Padma was also ragged. She was given an eraser and asked to measure the area of the 'Hawa Mahal'. Nonetheless, the seniors asked her to stop midway. Some girls were asked to take sips of the "GMC cola" which was a concoction of dal, coca cola, Fanta, tea, and coffee. While some girls were asked to dance, and some were asked to enact an ad for lingerie.

The hostel food was bad, but Padma had to make peace with it for her breakfast and sometimes dinner. Lunch was sent by her grandmother. She thanked the famous *Dabba* system of Bombay for she could relish her grandmother's delicious food every day. The concept of the *dabbawalas* goes way back to 1890 when Mahadeo Havaji Bachche started a lunch delivery service in Bombay with about a hundred men. This system is so good that Harvard School did a case study on them. Padma was in awe of their work efficiency. The dabbas had no name or address on them but were identified only with some numbers and colour coding. These men in white kurta pyjamas with a white cap would go about their daily activities so meticulously that they would hardly misplace a dabba.

The first six months were busy adjusting to the new environment, classes, ragging, and making new friends. The year and a half of the first MBBS just flew by. It was when they had to dissect the dead bodies which smelt so strongly of formalin. The dissection class was invariably before lunch break. Back then students didn't have the luxury of wearing gloves. The bare hands smelled so badly of the stench of formalin which couldn't be removed even with soap and water. Initially, it was difficult to eat after class but soon the students got used to it.

Padma had made a lot of new friends and got used to the hostel life. The weekends were spent with her Grandparents and the holidays with her family in Pune. Soon the months of the first MBBS came to an end which culminated in the first MBBS exams. One had to pass it to be promoted to the second MBBS. In the second MBBS, however, one could keep terms and take those exams in the final year.

One and half years of the Second MBBS were the days that all students look forward to. It's when they get to actually go to the wards and come in contact with the patients which is called the clinical posting. It was when they were taught to give injections, withdraw blood, listen to the sounds of the heart and the lungs, check the vital parameters, and so on. Padma smiled as she remembered a hilarious moment during the clinical posting of Gynaecology and Obstetrics. It was the first time their batch was to witness a delivery. They were a group of young budding doctors surrounding the first-time mother who was screaming in pain. Then suddenly they heard someone fall down. No! It wasn't the baby but one of their colleagues. Their friend who could not withstand the screams of the mother and the sight of blood fainted. The whole batch was busy taking care of him, just then they heard the cries of the new-born. Alas, they all had just missed the moment of witnessing a normal delivery.

The second year of MBBS was full of excitement and new happenings. It was the year when students were put in new batches according to their surnames. It was the year when new bonds were made and love blossomed. Now they could wear the doctor's white coats with a stethoscope around their neck and feel like a real doctor. One could call it the "happy year". Padma too had found her soulmate. Padma not only enjoyed the various clinical postings but looked forward to learning new things. One and half years rolled by so fast and the final year had already arrived. It was the crucial next one and a half years of the third MBBS that mattered. It would determine the specialisation they would get into. It also meant a lot of hard work. Specialising in Anaesthesia was Padma's second choice. She always wanted to do Obstetrics and Gynaecology but changed her mind after doing a temporary post for one month. Obstetrics was not her cup of tea.

After the initial uncertainty, everyone seemed to get the specialty they wanted.

Chapter Seven

Postgraduate Days

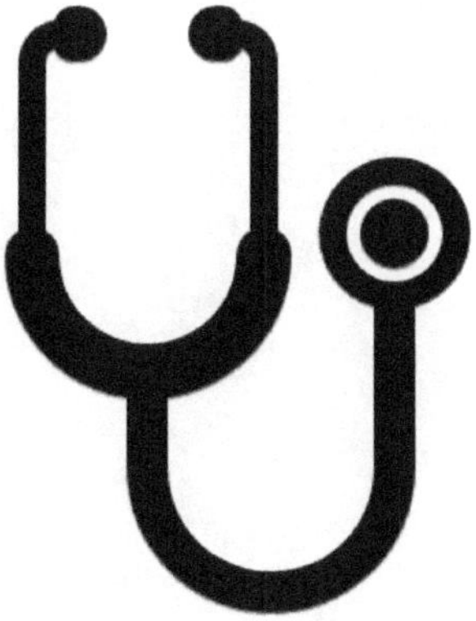

Padma joined the JJ group of hospitals again and she was looking forward to it. Although the initial days in the department were dramatic, she soon settled down in the department and started enjoying the daily routine. She looked forward to the mornings in the operation theatres. Operation theatres (O.T.) usually become a second home for an anaesthesiologist. Padma had to report by 7:30 am to the O.T. every day. On the first day, Padma was very apprehensive. Padma was posted in the general surgery O.T. She reached there before time and waited in the lobby of the O.T. Sister Janaki, the O.T. in-charge, looked at Padma and asked, "What's your name? You can wait in the female doctors' changing room." Sister Janaki was a tall slim lady in her forties. She seemed friendly and had a pleasant smile. After a while Sister came into the ladies changing room and gave instructions to all the newcomers asking them to change into the green O.T. dress. She spoke with authoritarian importance and Padma felt a little intimidated lest she knew that one day the anaesthesiologist and nurses would ultimately become best of friends.

In the coming days of the posting, the ladies changing room revealed itself like a pandora's box of stories. It was a room one would meet a lot of aspiring and established lady doctors. There would be consultants, the head of departments, and of course resident doctors. It was a place where the anaesthesiologists would order their morning breakfast as they would clock in early. They planned to eat it after they had started and settled their first case only to know that many times it would already be eaten up by the surgeons. It was also the place for gossip. Padma remembered once when a senior consultant lady surgeon had asked Sister Janaki to help her with the blouse back buttons and matter of fact smiling naughtily said, "Ladies, you need to teach your boyfriend or husband to do it."

Anaesthesiologist were basically in charge of all the operation theatres and emergency wards. Anesthesia was one of the busiest specialties but Padma loved her work. She was anesthetizing patients and saving lives too. An Anaesthesiologist would feel the thrill and an adrenaline rush every time a patient was put to sleep. They would titrate the doses of drugs so that the patient doesn't feel the pain during the surgery and then tactfully wake up the patient out of the anaesthetic slumber. It was also necessary that the patient is completely paralyzed and is not aware of the events during his surgery. All this was achieved by the anaesthesiologist who meticulously injected the drugs in their required doses. Padma was getting to learn a lot and was also learning the tricks of the trade!!

It was a known fact that at times the surgeons and the anaesthesiologist would be at loggerheads. The Surgeons usually thought that they were a superior breed and could order the anaesthesiologists around. The commonest dialogue that one could hear in the

O.T. was the surgeon telling the anaesthesiologist, "The patient is too tight. I need more relaxation. Do something." The anaesthesiologist would ignore it as the top-up muscle relaxation drug would have been just then injected. But the surgeon's ranting would continue. The senior anaesthesiologist and the junior would exchange meaningful glances to use their trick. The junior would then inject sterile distilled water instead of a drug to satisfy the surgeon and miraculously the surgeon would be happy with the relaxation. Let's call it the "Placebo surgeon effect".

Padma was posted in different specialties' operation theatres. Padma would always be empathetic towards her patients. She would dwell on their background and would take efforts to know them better during her preoperative rounds. Her seniors had warned her not to get emotionally attached to the patients. It could hurt her sometimes. That's exactly what happened.

Padma had to meet this lovely little girl several times who was scheduled for heart surgery. She had developed a special bond with the 3-year-old. This child was being postponed as she was not strong enough to withstand the major surgery. At last, she got the fitness and the day dawned for her to have the heart surgery. Padma was in the team of anaesthesiologists assigned to this case. She was excited but apprehensive as well. The surgery did go well and the recovery from anaesthesia was also good.

Padma thanked God as she accompanied the patient to the recovery room. She was then shifted to the ICCU. Padma made it a point to see her again before she retired for the day. The next morning Padma left for the OT early so that she could check on the child before her routine cases. As she entered the ICCU full of hope she got the shocking news that the child had died the previous night because of complications. Padma could not hold back her tears and was very depressed. She found the parents of the child waiting outside the ICCU. It pained to see their solemn faces and teary eyes. When Padma approached them, the mother burst out crying. Padma hugged her and tried to console her but in vain. The father then got up and with folded hands said, "All doctors had tried their best to give a new lease of life to my daughter and I thank all of you. But God had different plans for her. He loved her so much that he called her back soon. We will always remember you for the joy you gave my daughter for the past month. She always looked forward to your visits to the ward." Padma was overwhelmed. Even in this hour of sorrow, they did not forget to thank the doctors. Medicine is not all about curing but the art of providing relief by patiently listening to your patients.

The scenario of the 21st century has completely changed. Here the patients and their relatives are just finding some reason to bash the doctors in the hospital or sue them. One must understand that no doctor would want to let his patient die. Medicine is a complicated science and no doctor is God. Doctors try their level best to improve the condition of their patients. They forgo their meals, and their sleep to render their expert services but sometimes it is beyond their capability, and as the father rightly said, "God has other plans."

Feeling depressed and contrite, Padma couldn't get the face of the little girl out of her thoughts. It was a while before Padma could come out of her self-imposed mental exile. She remembered what her seniors had told her about not getting too attached to the patients but then wasn't it worth the time she spent with the child as the child had yearned for her company too and they had spent some happy moments together. Padma decided to listen to her heart and continued to be caring and empathetic towards her patients.

Her Residency days in the department of anaesthesia were full of interesting cases. Be it a hectic call at the casualty or emergency calls from the various departments, it was as usual a busy emergency for Padma. She had just finished an interesting case in the paediatric operation theatre. The surgery had gone on for five long hours. Padma was tired but she had no time to rest. She was called immediately to the casualty. There had been a road traffic accident. The man was bleeding and gasping for breath. Padma quickly assessed him. He needed to be intubated, that is to put a tube in his windpipe to secure his airway.

His mouth was full of blood. She looked at the man. He looked pale and was barely conscious. Padma did not bother with her hands getting messy with the blood and successfully secured the patient's airway and connected him to oxygen. With the primarily required interventions she could stabilise the patient and the surgeon who was already trying to assess the injuries could start his treatment.

Padma heard her stomach growling and that is when she realised that she hadn't eaten her lunch. It was already five in the evening. She decided to rush up to the fifth-floor canteen commonly called the FFC and grab something to eat. When she was near the lift, she saw the ward boy rushing towards her. He was a short plum man dressed in white shirt and white trousers with a heavy ledger in his hands. It was an emergency on call register. Padma looked at the register as she was the chief resident anaesthesiologist on call that day. That meant she was responsible for all the emergencies and had to decide which resident doctor to send for which call based on their capability. But as always, her on-call day was so busy that she had no one to spare for the latest emergency case. She signed the register and decided to attend the case herself.

He was a patient in the ICCU. As the ICCU was on the fifth floor, Padma went to do a preoperative assessment for the patient before heading to the FFC. The cardiologist told her that it was a very critical case and the patient might not survive. He needed a below

-the-knee amputation because of gangrene. He was so sick with a bad heart and uncontrolled diabetes that Padma asked her senior to be present for the case. There was some time till the orthopaedic OT would be ready for the case. Padma rushed to the FFC to pick up a packet of biscuits. She ate them on the way to the ICCU. Her Senior was already at the ICCU when she arrived there. They decided to shift the patient to the operation theatre. Padma was on the head end of the trolley on which the patient lay and was holding the mask to give oxygen to him. As they reached the entrance of the operation theatre the patient gasped and vomited. Padma's hands were soiled with vomitus. The ECG monitor showed a flat line. She just wiped her hands with the trolley sheet while trying to revive the patient as they moved him into the recovery area of the operation theatre. The attending cardiologist also helped them but in vain. They all knew that this outcome was a high possibility but when a life is lost there is always a void created. The feeling of helplessness and making peace with the limits of their profession was palpable.

Chapter Eight

Marriage On Cards

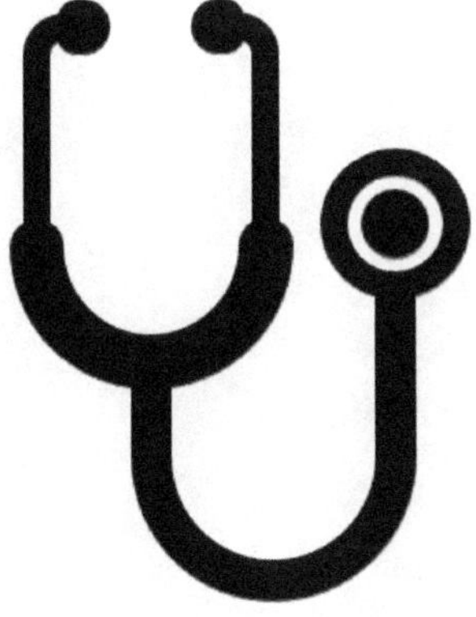

Padma was very committed to her work but she also had a personal life. Ram and she had known each other for 4 years. Talks of marriage were doing the rounds. It was the internship year for Padma. The internship is the year after the doctors have passed their final MBBS exam. It involves working six months in the hospital they studied in and six months in a rural hospital. Rural posting meant some time off and that meant Padma could spend time with her family in Pune. She looked forward to meeting her parents, grandmother, and sister. It was one such visit that the talks about marriage began.

Padma boarded the train to Pune. She hadn't informed her family that she was coming. She wanted to surprise them. Padma was waiting at the V.T. railway station. It was the first stop. As the train approached the station, Padma, who had been running on the platform along with the train, got into the ladies' compartment. She managed to get her favourite seat, a single seat next to the window on the upper deck. This train, the Sinhagad Express, was a double-decker train. It was a convenient train as she would reach Pune by 7:00 pm and she could be at home by 7:30 pm.

Padma settled herself in the cosy corner and managed to take a nap for an hour. The train reached Pune on time so she could get the bus home quickly. She alighted at her stop and as she walked home, she felt so happy. Padma rang the bell at the front door. It was already dark. Her mother opened the door and the surprised look on her mother's face was something to capture on the camera. Padma's mother was very happy to see her. Her youngest sister came running down from the bedroom and hugged her. Padma was the eldest of three sisters. The sister younger than her was now in the US pursuing her master's degree.

Her grandmother said, "Padma, you must be tired and hungry. Why don't you freshen up and have dinner? You sisters can catch up later."

Just then the doorbell rang. It was her father. He too was surprised and of course, like a concerned father said, "You could have called us up. I would have come to pick you up."

Padma smiled and said, "But I wanted to surprise you all." Padma and her sister talked till late into the night.

It was already 8 :00 am by the time Padma woke up in the morning. When she went down to have her cup of tea Padma's father was having his breakfast. "Good morning, Padma. Did you sleep well?" Padma's father asked.

Padma said, "We were talking till late, and later I had a sound sleep. When will you be back from work?"

After her father had left for work, she went into the kitchen. She heard her mother giving instructions to the servants. Her mother asked, "What do you want to have for lunch dear? Will you have scrambled eggs and toast for breakfast? When do you have to go back?"

Padma was always pampered when she came home. She smiled and hugged her mother and said, "I will eat whatever you make. After all, home food is always comforting food. I will be here for a week." Padma after her bath had a good breakfast and then spent some time in the garden. They had two gardeners but it was her mother who supervised their gardening. Padma's mother had managed to plant a beautiful bed of roses with fifteen varieties of roses, one of them being a black rose. After spending some time in the garden when it started to get hot, Padma came in and went to the kitchen to make herself a glass of lime juice. Her mother was already making preparations for lunch. Padma's father would come home around 1 to 1 :30 pm for lunch and then they could have lunch together.

The aroma in the kitchen was already making her hungry. Padma's mother looked at her and slowly broached the topic of marriage. Padma was taken unaware when her mother said, "Padma, your uncle in the USA has asked if you would be open to settling down in the USA. His friend's son is a neurologist there and your uncle knows the family well. But if you want to stay back in India then your Andheri Aunt too has a proposal for you. The boy is a doctor who has an established practice in Bombay. The family is also known to her."

This sudden onslaught of information left Padma with no choice but to reveal the secret she had kept for the last 4 years. Padma slowly said, "Mummy, I have to tell you something. I am in love with a boy in my class and we want to get married. He is a Tamilian."

Her mother looked at her and asked, "What about his family? South Indians are very conservative people. Will they accept a girl from another community? If you are sure you want to spend the rest of your life with him, we would like to meet him. But remember dear that it is not only the boy you marry but you marry into a family and that may mean a lot of adjustments. The culture, the food, the language, everything will be different."

Padma felt a bit apprehensive after the conversation. She said, "Mummy, he is close to his sister and has already told her. Since his father is no more his brother-in-law will have a say in the matter. I think his mother has her own apprehensions. Yes, it's going to be a little difficult at his end but he is sure that he will be able to convince all of them."

After dinner, that night Padma's parents had a lengthy talk with her regarding this matter and Padma's father said he would like to meet Ram. Her parents were open-minded people and were confident that Padma's choice would be right. When Padma got back to Bombay, she was pleasantly surprised to learn that Ram had also talked to his family and that his brother-in-law wanted to meet her. The meeting was scheduled after two days. Padma was already nervous but was also eager to meet his side of the family.

Ram and Padma sat on either side of Ram's brother-in-law and after the customary greetings, the serious conversation started. He said, "Padma you are not a South Indian and so Ram's mother is a little sceptical about how you would fit in. She feels that a daughter-in-law from their culture would look after her well and will be able to adjust better in the new family." Padma smiled but the next statement really startled her. He continued and said, "We could change Ram's mind to marry a girl of our choice."

She immediately retaliated without thinking of the consequences. Padma said, "I am sure you cannot change Ram's mind. Anyway, I wouldn't marry a person who is not sure of his feelings. I can understand the apprehensions of Ram's mother but as far as the topic of a girl from your community being more suitable, can you give a guarantee for that?" Padma wondered if she had been rude but she was happy that she had spoken her mind. Anyway, things turned out fine in the end. After talks between the families, Padma and Ram were married in Pune with the blessings of elders in the third year of her anaesthesia residency. It was a South Indian Tamil Brahmin wedding and Padma's side of the family enjoyed it thoroughly.

Chapter Nine

The Newly Married

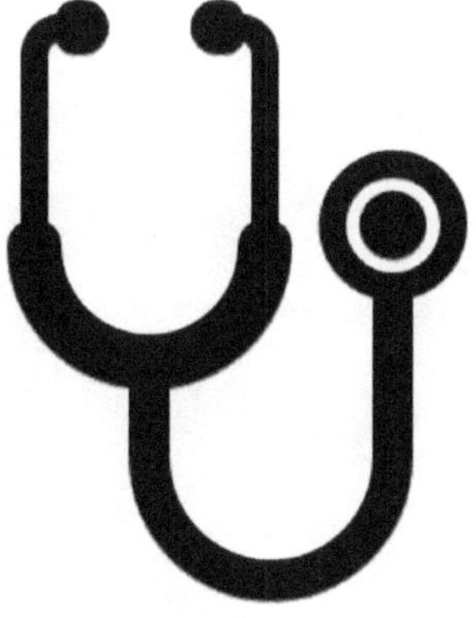

After the fifteen days of leave which were full of festivities of the marriage and the bliss of a short honeymoon, Padma and Ram were back to work. Padma was a chief resident now and that meant more responsibilities and a rotation in the major postings like the cardiac and neurology specialties. It also meant a lot of hard work and erratic timings. One had to find time to study as it was the last year of residency and the final exams were around the corner. Padma was also adjusting to her new family. She was pleasantly surprised that she was able to gel with her mother-in-law well. She was also getting used to eating a different kind of cuisine. Now her "Dabba" was sent by her mother-in-law, "Amma". It was completely different from Padma's mother's food. She was intrigued to know that South Indian food went beyond the customary Dosa, Idli, and Sambar. She greatly appreciated the efforts taken by Amma to pack two different Dabbas for Ram and her. Amma was very accommodating when Padma would visit home on the weekends. Padma looked forward to the weekends. Home visits were interlaced with yummy South Indian food, learning about the family and the extended family when Amma would tell Padma interesting stories about the family. Padma too introduced her family connections to Amma.

Padma's new home was a 2-bedroom flat in Thane. It was typically a Tamil Brahmin household. You would be greeted with a beautifully done Rangoli outside the main door. Then there was the living cum dining room on the left and the kitchen on the right. Although it was a small kitchen, as all Tamil Brahmin households would have, considerable space was dedicated to the pooja. The pooja area had been carefully organised to make space for photos and idols of gods. It felt so serene and peaceful. The kitchen also had numerous shelves and cupboards to stack all the kitchen items. Actually, there were so many inbuilt cupboards in the whole house to keep your things that the house was organised well. This is something one can learn from the houses in Mumbai where space is a constraint. Even a small flat would look spacious because of the clever organisation ideas.

 Padma also loved to shop for her little niece, Ram's sister's daughter. These gifts Amma would take along with her when she visited her daughter in Bangalore. She was also trying to understand the Tamil language. Of course, her husband had taught her one sentence which meant "Don't talk in Tamil. I don't understand Tamil". But Padma was determined to learn the language and the culture eventually. The timeline was questionable because she could meet Amma only on the weekends. Also, the three of them usually conversed in Hindi.

Final exams were around the corner. There was hardly any time for "me time" for Padma. In fact, she could get very little quality time with Ram. Super specialty postings at the J.J Hospital meant that Padma had to clock in early and there was no end time. She would be so tired when she would reach the G.T Hospital, one of the hospitals in the JJ group of hospitals, where Ram was posted that Padma wouldn't even have the energy to have dinner. Ram suggested that she stayed back at the J.J hostel till her major postings were over. Was Ram being sarcastic? But with the present circumstances, it seemed to be the best option. They could meet on the weekends, Padma thought. Work was as hectic as possible.

 Being the chief resident meant a lot of responsibilities and busy schedules. As usual, Padma's emergencies were as busy as ever. On one such emergency duty, Padma had to attend the emergency surgery O.T. at 1:00 am. She knew this was a critical case not only because of the severity of the injuries but also because of the people involved in it. It was a case of a gang war between the two famous underworld gangs in which two men, one from each gang were seriously injured. When Padma reached the emergency O.T. She saw a huge crowd outside the operation theatre. The policemen were trying desperately to control the crowd which also involved keeping the people of both gangs separate. Emotions were running high and that meant the situation could turn violent anytime. Padma felt a sense of relief when she saw her Senior walking towards the operation theatre. They both entered the operation theatre amidst police security. The patients were already inside. Padma did a quick assessment of the patients. Her juniors had already taken care of the prerequisites for the cases. Both patients were on the table. The patients were in critical condition. The injuries were so grievous and they were bleeding profusely from the gunshot wounds. Blood was being given to them as they had lost a lot of blood. The situation was like a double edge sword. They had to save both patients but if one of them died on the table the mob could turn violent. Padma's fears came true. They could not save one of the patients. Padma's senior and Padma consulted the police. After a quick discussion and deliberation, the police requested the team of doctors not to declare table death. There were not enough police personnel to handle the situation. So, Padma and her team decided to shift both patients to the ICU- intensive care unit ventilating them on the way that is pumping oxygen through the tube in the mouth. Then they would tell the dead patient's gang that their member was critical and declare death after one hour. They hoped that this would help the gang to prepare their minds and prevent a violent outcome. With God's grace, the night passed through smoothly.

Work was as busy as ever and soon it was time to go on study leave. Padma was overwhelmed with the overload of work and the pressure of studying for the finals. She just wanted to get away from the mad routine. She and Ram decided to go to Marine Drive, one of the famous tourist spots in Bombay. The evening sun was just setting in, giving a beautiful golden hue to the sea. The gentle cool sea breeze was very refreshing. Ram and Padma sat on the embankment facing the sea. There was a steady stream of people walking and talking on the footpath but the cacophony of their voices somehow seemed to fade in the noise of the waves hitting the rocks. Padma felt relaxed. She tried to freeze her thoughts and not think about work or the final exams.

Chapter Ten

Exam Leave

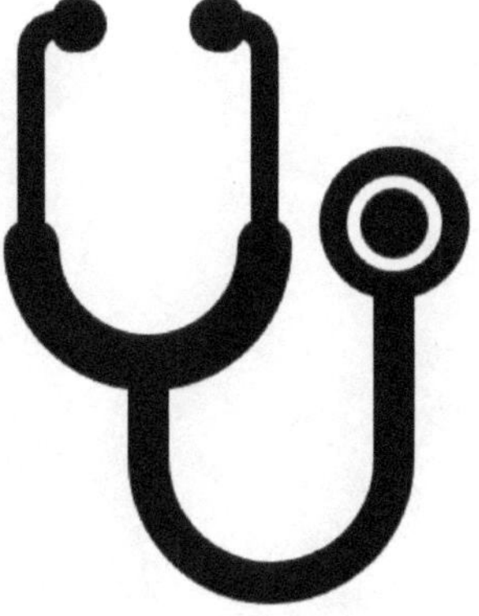

The final exams were scheduled in the month of January. Their batch would be on exam leave from the next month, that is the month of November.

Padma and Ram were busy preparing for their exams. Padma's room was on the 7th floor of the newly constructed building for the resident doctors. It was actually a luxury to have a room with an attached bathroom and an intercom facility. Ram had also shifted all his luggage to her room. Now Amma sent the Dabba to Padma's hostel with enough food for both of them. Padma had a small hotplate with few vessels. She had a little stock of rice, dal, tea, coffee, and milk powder. If they didn't feel like eating in the canteen, Padma would make some khichdi.

They would study in the library. The library was occupied by the exam-going batch till 2:00 am. Padma also visited the department to clear some doubts and meet her guide. She managed to do the thesis submission in time after the customary process of proofreading, typing, making photocopies, and then binding. It was a difficult process compared to how it is done now. Back then without the computer, thesis completion was an ordeal. One had to first manually write the content. The required photographs had to be clicked on the camera and then develop them. Once the manuscript was approved by the guide it had to be typed. There were designated places near the V.T. station where all the postgraduates would get their thesis typed by a typist. Once the typing was done the main copy had to be photocopied to get a total of four sets. Then these sets had to be bound. Typically, it would have to be a hard binding with a black cover. The photographs which were developed were then pasted on the required pages. Oh my God, a long process indeed.

Ram was an early riser. He would wake up in the morning around 3:30 a m and start studying. Padma slept late and studied with her friends who stayed on the same floor. The exam study routine was set for everyone. The 7th floor of the resident doctors' quarters had all exam-going postgraduates. In the evenings to break the monotony and the tension of studying, some of them would meet on the terrace. The cool evening sea breeze would be refreshing. One could see only tall buildings around. The sky would have a hue of golden colour cast by the setting sun. The birds could be seen flying back to their nests. One could gaze down to see the streets beyond the gates of the campus with people running to catch the bus back home. The streets surrounding the campus would be bursting with diverse people going about their own activities oblivious to race, religion, and caste which was never a matter of concern in the city called Bombay. It was a safe city even late in the night except for certain areas. It was customary for many of the doctors to go for a walk across the street after the library hours at 2:00 am to have a glass of juice from the "Sapna juice centre" or a glass of hot piping milk from the stall on the street. Abdul Chacha would give special glasses of milk with extra cream on the top especially for the doctors. Then there was the "Almas Hotel" famous for its caramel custard. Food was never a problem in Bombay with so many road side eateries selling good cheap food. There was the famous "Parsi dairy" Kulfi and "Kayani Bakery"near the G.T Hospital. Kayani Bakery was famous for its Bun Maska and tea. The watermelon slush was also something to relish there. Padma and Ram also loved the peach melba ice cream at the "Badshah ice cream parlour" near the Crawford market.

Mumbai is home to many cultures and the Iranian Zoroastrian culture is one of the founding spirits of Bombay. In the 19th and 20th centuries, many Irani immigrants settled in the city, led by the path of their Parsi cousins who came to India 1200 years before them. The Iranians settled here and set up their businesses and Kyani and Co were one of them. Founded in 1904 by Mr Khodram. Kyani & Co started as a bakery that made bread, biscuits, cakes and other tea time bakes. It has stood the test of time and still gives you the nostalgic feeling of the bygone era.

Parsi Dairy Farm, a family business, was established in 1916. It was started by a young Parsi entrepreneur, the Late Nariman Ardeshir. The signature Parsi Dairy Farm "Malai Kulfi", its soft and airy "Sutarfeni", the bright orange "Dudh Badam Halwa", the melt-in-your-mouth milk drops and Full-Fat Milk can still be purchased.

It also held a special place in Padma's life. During her early school days when she visited her grandparents' place, Parsi Diary was a place that she frequented with her aunts and Uncles. There was a hilarious episode associated with Parsi Dairy Ice Cream which Padma had told Ram on their first visit there. It so happened that during one of the customary summer vacation visits to her grandparents' place Padma's Aunts and Uncles took her to Parsi Dairy. They all ate ice cream. As she had a mild cough her uncle told her not to tell her mother that she had eaten ice cream. After reaching home Padma's mother asked her, "Did you have fun?" Padma replied with a smile, "I had lots of fun. We went to the beach and ate "bhel" and very innocently looking at her aunt said, "but did not have any ice cream." Immediately everyone burst out laughing. After all, the lie was exposed. Padma started crying. Her mother hugged her and said, "It's okay. We will drink some hot water now."

Exam preparations were going on in full swing. By the end of November, the exam tension in the exam-going batch was obvious. All had made plans for their future. Some would be applying for super specialisation, some had planned to fly to greener pastures, some wanted to do a fellowship. For some, marriage was on cards. All were looking forward to this new phase in their life. Other than the exam preparations life was peaceful. They no longer had the hectic schedule of a resident doctor. The only thing on their mind was to clear the exam.

Lest they knew that everything was to change in the month of December. A storm was brewing and all were going to get caught in that. And so did it happen. Their routine was turned upside down on December 6, 1992.

Chapter Eleven

Babri Masjid Demolition

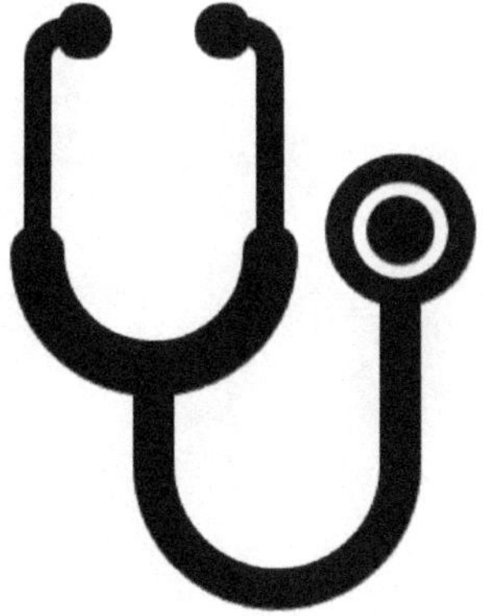

Padma speaks…

It was a routine day for everyone. Ram as usual had got up early to study. At 6.00 am he woke me up. He made coffee for both of us. The coffee was refreshing. I had already made my study timetable the previous day and planned to stick to it. After all, there were not many days left for the final exams.

Around lunch time, the rumours of riots that were doing rounds were confirmed. All Department heads were instructed to call back the exam-going batch for duty. My batch mates and I were asked to assemble at the department on the 6th floor. The meeting was quickly conducted and the batch was told to be on call. We were briefed on the situation.

The communal riots had broken out after the demolition of the Babri Masjid throughout the country. The situation was volatile and grim. All the doctors were needed on a war footing. The emergency department that had a trickle of casualties was now overflowing. There seemed to be total chaos in the main building of the JJ Hospital. Similar situations also prevailed in the other 3 peripheral hospitals. The doctors were asked not to leave the campus. All the gates were closed except the main gate to the hospital.

I stepped hesitantly onto the ground floor of the JJ hospital. There were people everywhere. It was not new for JJ Hospital to be crowded but today it felt different. Relatives were rushing their near and dear ones towards the casualty room oblivious of what was happening around them. There were doctors with their white coats and stethoscopes around their necks also rushing around taking care of the patients.

Someone tapped on my shoulder. I looked back. It was my colleague. "We are needed in the casualty. Come let's rush," he said.

When we reached the casualty, the scenario was worse. The police were trying to control the crowd but in vain. People were running helter-skelter. A sense of desperation and anger could be seen on their faces. Just then there was a tug on my coat. As I looked behind, I saw a young lady crying. She had an infant in her arms. Her saree and hands were stained with blood. Her dirty face and ruffled hair told you that she was from the streets. Even before I could ask her about her predicament, the lady between her sobs pointed towards a man lying on the floor in a pool of blood and begged with folded hands, "Please help my husband. They have stabbed him with a sword." I bent down towards the man to feel his pulse. He was barely alive. His pulse was weak. He had lost a lot of blood. I immediately put a cannula in his vein so that I could give him some fluids till they could get blood to infuse and stabilise him and take him up for surgery. I looked at the lady. She seemed to be a little relieved. I told her, "Doctors are doing their best to save the patients. Please pray and have faith in God."

Mayhem that the riots had unleashed was beyond imagination. I thought, "How can a man turn against his own brethren? How can neighbours who were once friends become enemies? Is it really happening?" So many questions just came flooding into my mind.

There were many more patients like that lady's husband who needed immediate attention. The situation was overwhelming. There were people everywhere. The stench of blood and other body fluids interlaced with the smell of spirit was nauseating. But in this situation, one's senses just would go numb. I heard the senior nurse in charge call out my name. It was sister Janaki. As she approached me, I could see the serious and sad expression on her face. She pulled me to a corner and said, "Dr. Padma, we have a dicey situation. There are so many coming in with serious injuries. We are running short of blood. Some cases are unsalvageable. You anaesthetists need to examine them and make the decision regarding which patient to shift to the operation theatre."

I gave her a stern look and said, "Don't make us play God. Who are we to decide who lives and who dies? We are here to save lives. This is ridiculous."

Sister Janaki said, "Don't get emotional. We have no choice. We are short of resources and we have to use the limited resources we have to save a patient who has a better chance of survival. These are orders from the higher authorities."

I couldn't comprehend what was happening and stood there dumbfounded. But there was no time to waste. We all quickly organised ourselves and then the emergency room worked like a well-oiled machine. We decided to prioritise the patients unlike normal times on the survival rate rather than on the severity of injuries. There were a lot of casualties too. I also heard that the Morgue was soon going to run out of space.

The day ended very late for me. I was exhausted both physically and mentally. I came back to my room and had a hot water bath. Ram asked me if I wanted to eat anything but I had lost my appetite. I just wanted to unwind. "What could be a better place than the terrace," I thought. The sun had already set. Ram and I reached the terrace only to find that there were so many resident doctors already there. They all look worried, distraught, and exhausted. My friend called out from the other end of the terrace and said, "Padma, look around. This can't be happening."

I was aghast to see that some of the buildings were on fire. The light from the fires illuminated the dark skies. The blaring sound of the fire engines could be heard distinctly. Suddenly some of the doctors started to congregate at one corner. They were all looking down cautiously. We too joined them. I just could not believe my eyes when I saw some people pulling up the shutters of some of the shops below only to remove a bundle of swords to distribute it to the crowd waiting outside. It was inconceivable. We had seen a lot of patients with sword injuries. Some injuries were so gruesome indicating the sword had been swirled inside after stabbing, ensuring the person died. I could take it no more and ran back to my room. I just wanted to sleep and wished this was just a bad dream but sleep evaded me.

The Government had declared a curfew in most of the areas of Bombay. Everything was suspended including the train services. Bombay now had a deserted look. The police were given a free hand to shoot at sight. Now the casualty room was filled with patients who had bullet wounds. In spite of the curfew, some mobs had dared to defy the orders and create unrest. But the situation was brought under control and the train services resumed. Ram was worried about his mother and decided to pay her a visit and be back in 2 days. Although I was worried about the situation after the riots, it was necessary for Ram to check on Amma. I had lots to study and so I stayed back.

Chapter Twelve

Second Riots

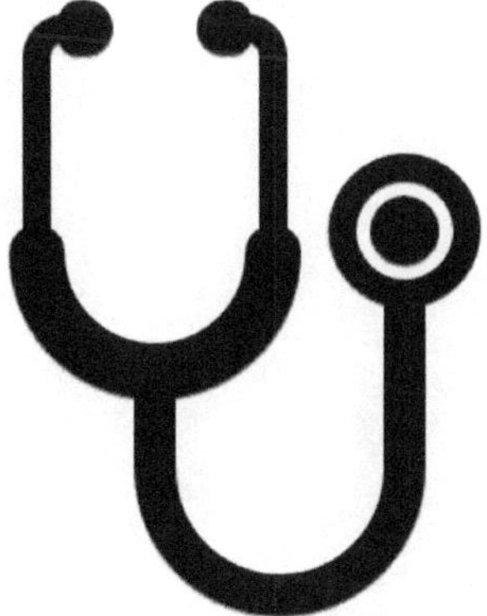

Padma speaks……

I was busy studying. It was 2 days since Ram had left for home. I was awaiting his return when there was a knock on the door. I expectantly opened the door only to find the ward boy with a circular in his hand. He asked me to sign it. "What is it?" I asked. He looked at me blankly. I read the circular and had a sick feeling in my stomach. This can't be true, I thought. The second riots had started and all of us were asked to come back to duty again. Oh God! Ram was to come today. I hoped he had not started. I was immersed in my thoughts when the ward boy called, "Doctor please sign the circular. I have to get the signatures from other doctors too." I quickly signed it and closed the door. As soon as I could gather my thoughts, I rushed down to the ground floor to make a call to Ram. I was pleasantly relieved to hear his voice. Before I could talk, he told me that he couldn't come as the train services were suspended. I breathed a sense of relief and asked him to stay put at home till the situation improved.

I went back to my room and as I opened the door, I heard the intercom ring. I knew it had to be from the department. I was asked to report to the plastic surgery operation theatre and take charge of it. I donned my doctor's coat, put my stethoscope around my neck, and walked quickly towards the department. I could see a large number of people who had gathered there. There were also some policemen trying to control the crowd. As I reached the department and climbed up the stairs under police protection I was scared for my life. The policeman opened the age-old iron shutters which had stood the test of time I hoped. He let me in and quickly closed it behind me preventing the crowd from entering the operation theatre. As I moved in, I could hear some of the people banging on the shutter and shouting, "We want to talk to the lady doctor." I turned back and looked at their angry faces. The policeman told me not to talk to them but I gathered some courage and answered their queries. As I approached them and stood across the barrier of the shutter some of them shouted angrily, "You all are government doctors and are hand in glove with the government. See how they have shot our people. You are the doctor to give anaesthesia and what if you choose not to get them out of anaesthesia and ensure they die because the police couldn't kill them." I just couldn't believe what I had heard. There was so much mistrust in the doctors who were working round the clock to save lives. "The circumstances had made these people insane," I thought. I gathered my composure and answered them, "Doctors are working hard to save lives. When we work, we are beyond the constraints of the boundaries created by religion, politics, or personal opinions. So be assured all the patients will be given utmost care."

I didn't wait for their response and rushed to the operation theatre after donning my gown, cap, and mask. There was no time to waste. We had a quick discussion with the surgeons and the police and after deliberation with my team, I decided to use the anaesthetic drug which would give good pain relief but only a light state of hypnosis ensuring that the patient recovered quickly. We neither had enough space in the recovery room nor did we have the time to keep the patients after surgery for a long time. My team was excellent and I assigned roles to each of the team members. We tried not to jump roles unless really necessary. The surgeons also did their bit very efficiently. There was always a policeman to collect the bullets as they were removed. The whole thing was exhausting both mentally and physically. After the good recovery of the first few patients, the crowd outside sobered down and also thanked us. I thanked my stars for not being posted in the casualty this time as I couldn't have faced the death of many innocent beings at close quarters again.

I was very tired when I reached my room late at night. I had a hot water bath and made some tea for myself. I had no appetite to eat anything. As I sipped my tea, I thought about the day's events only to feel depressed and helpless. I missed Ram so much and wondered how he was coping at home. I must have dozed off studying on my bed only to be woken up by the morning sun. Though it was another day, the same routine followed.

We were all running out of food supplies. Most of the Canteens had closed down. Although the curfew was relaxed for a few hours of the day, no one dared venture out as everyone felt unsafe. Even the Ambulances were not spared in some places. It seemed like people had lost their senses. It was difficult to imagine that a place like Bombay where people from all walks of life, of different religions, castes and creeds co-existed peacefully had suddenly turned into a war zone with no value for life. I wondered who was behind all this insanity. There were speculations that it was triggered by external sources who were on a mission to disrupt the harmony in India.

As I got ready to report back to duty there was a knock on the door. "I hope it's not the ward boy with another circular, "I thought as I opened the door. My happiness knew bounds when I saw Ram at the door. But I was surprised and curious to know how he had managed to reach JJ Hospital. When Ram told me about his heroic adventure, I was not only frightened but also angry because he had taken such a big risk. He had managed to take the early morning train from Thane to VT station. There were very few trains plying on various train routes. Ram decided to catch the early train lest the next one got cancelled. After he got off the train at VT Station which was the last stop, he quickly walked to the St George hospital. Of course, he carried his doctor's ID in case one of the policemen asked questions. When he reached the hospital, he made inquiries if there would be an Ambulance going to JJ Hospital. To his luck, one was to leave in half an hour in which he managed to get a lift.

I had tears in my eyes and was also very overwhelmed. "Do you know what risk you have taken? You could have been attacked on the train or when you were walking. Even the Ambulances are not spared. Were you out of your senses to embark on such a journey?" I shouted. "Please go and call up Amma that you have reached safely. She must be very worried," I said.

The riots continued for some time with decreasing intensity. As the riots died down and the law and order was restored the Hospital had a herculean task of handing over the bodies to the relatives and disposing of the unclaimed ones. The Morgue was overflowing with them. Our exams were postponed and the exam-going batch was back on exam leave. But the impact of the riots had left a lasting impression on everyone and one could say it disabled us mentally. No one was in the mood to study anymore. We all wanted to just pass our exams and move on without taking these memories with us. It was not easy and made me question life itself. I wanted to forget all this and consider it a bad dream. Bombay was never the same after this. An evil eye was cast on my lovely city where I was born and reborn again. I could never make a home here I thought as I moved miles away to begin a new life...

About The Author

Dr. Pradnya Sriram is an Anaesthesiologist who is also the co-founder of her hospital Pradnya Nethralaya in Bangalore. She did her post-graduation in Anaesthesia from Grant Medical College Mumbai and has an experience of 30 years in this field. She is a Rotarian and also an alumnus of the Goldman Sachs 10000 women entrepreneurs initiative from IIM Bangalore.

Dr. Pradnya is a trainer for basic life support and has been instrumental in quality improvement in hospitals. She loves to read books, write, cook, and paint.